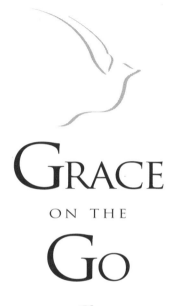

GRACE
ON THE
GO

Quick Prayers for Compassionate Caregivers

BARBARA BARTOCCI

MOREHOUSE PUBLISHING

An imprint of Church Publishing Incorporated
Harrisburg—New York

Unless otherwise noted, the Scripture quotations contained herein are from the New Revised Standard Version Bible, copyright © 1989 by the Division of Christian Education of the National Council of Churches of Christ in the U.S.A. Used by permission. All rights reserved.

Morehouse Publishing, 4775 Linglestown Road, Harrisburg, PA 17105

Morehouse Publishing, 445 Fifth Avenue, New York, NY 10016

Morehouse Publishing is an imprint of Church Publishing Incorporated.

Cover design by Jennifer Glosser

Library of Congress Cataloging-in-Publication Data

Bartocci, Barbara.
  Grace on the go : quick prayers for compassionate caregivers / Barbara Bartocci.
    p. cm.
  ISBN 978-0-8192-2286-2 (pbk.)
  1. Caregivers—Prayers and devotions. I. Title.
BV4910.9.B37 2008
242'.88—dc22

                                        2007037629

Printed in the United States of America

08 09 10 11 12 13   10 9 8 7 6 5 4 3 2 1

There are only four kinds of people in this world—those who have been caregivers, those who currently are caregivers, those who will be caregivers, and those who need caregivers.
—Former first lady Rosalynn Carter

I lay my "why?"
Before Your cross
In worship kneeling,
My mind beyond all hope,
My heart beyond all feeling,
And worshipping,
Realize that I
In knowing You,
Don't need a "Why?"
—Ruth Bell Graham

Trust in the Lord with all your heart
And do not rely on your own insight.
—Proverbs 3:5

CONTENTS

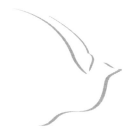

Chapter One
Beginnings

Helpless, I stared at the telephone, wondering what to do.

My mother had just called with dreadful news. "Barbara, the cancer has come back." She sounded frightened and fragile—not at all like my feisty, tough-minded mom. My father had died two years earlier, and I was their only daughter. My mother needed me. "Will you come?" she asked. Her voice quavered.

Of course I would go. But I was waiting for *my* only daughter to deliver her first baby. She was two days past her due date.

I knew Sony wanted me to be there for the birth. Should I leave at once for California to be with my mom? Or wait until the baby came? I felt so pulled by these two conflicting needs.

And I was apprehensive. Once I got there, how long could I afford to stay? Part of me said, "You'll stay as long as your mom needs you." I was a self-employed business writer, so I could set my own schedule. But another part of me worried, "How long can you afford to take time off from paying clients?"

After a lot of thought, I waited for my daughter to give birth, though another week passed before that happened. Three hours after my grandson was born, I was on a plane for California.

Later, I would learn that my dilemma and my worry reflected what many others feel. There are twenty-five million of us: one out of every twelve Americans is a family caregiver. If you're reading this, you're probably one of them. Relatives provide nearly eighty percent of all home health care, and most of us feel pretty overwhelmed.

And it's not just elderly parents we're caring for.

A young wife whose war-injured husband is permanently disabled cried softly, "I'm only twenty-three! I never expected something like this when we got married!"

The husband whose wife is in a wheelchair with MS might say the same. Or my friend whose mentally disabled adult son will always have to live with her.

When I was caring for my mom, I sometimes felt as if she

and I were on an island and everyone else lived across the water on the mainland. How could they possibly know what it was like for us?

Caregivers experience such continual rushes of adrenaline. Often, it's a daily roller coaster ride of hope and despair. There is the awful helplessness of watching someone you love drift into dementia or cry out in pain or angrily demand, "Why did you put me here?" And—let's be honest—most caregivers feel an occasional tug of resentment because this is *not* what you planned on doing with your life.

Prayer became one of my lifelines. Connecting to God through the suffering Christ helped me cope with stress that otherwise might have overwhelmed me. Recently I read that two-thirds of people who become caretakers say they rely heavily on prayer, and most feel that prayer helps.

In this book, you will read many caregivers' stories along with prayers that are written especially for you. You will also find, at the end of each chapter, what I call "Steps of Holy Action" because—have you noticed?—sometimes the Holy Spirit comes into our lives in very practical ways. You'll also learn how to turn individual caregiving tasks into sixty-second prayer opportunities.

Finally, because caregivers are always on the go, the book is sized so you can tuck it easily into your purse or pocket. Keep it with you. Read it in bits and pieces. Read it more than once. It is my devout hope it will help you find more of God's strengthening grace as you care for your loved one.

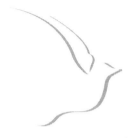

Chapter Two
Fear

My father was being prepped for open-heart surgery when my college-student son, Andy, telephoned him. "Granddaddy, I'll come see you tomorrow."

His grandfather chuckled. "Well, give me a day or two. This isn't a little Novocain job, you know." He was still chuckling as he related the conversation to me. I wondered: did I sense any anxiety in his voice? This was his second open-heart surgery. He put me at ease. "I'll be fine. Relieved to get it behind me."

But a few hours later, I knew it wasn't fine. My father had suffered a heart attack during surgery. Now he lay critically ill in the ICU.

There are many doors into the world of care-giving.

A cardio infarction like my dad's. A stroke. A fall . . . and you step through the door in an instant. Other times, it's more gradual. A chronic disease like multiple sclerosis. Alzheimer's. Cancer. . . .

By whatever door, the passage into care-giving changes lives. And no matter how willing you are—or how responsible—there are accompanying fears. You find yourself coming awake at 4 a.m. with questions clawing at your mind:

- What if I make the wrong decision?
- How can I bear my loved one's pain?
- Will I have enough money to do this?
- What if *I* get sick?

And, maybe not consciously asked, but in long-term care-giving, this very real question: "What about *me*? My dreams? My future? Must I give them up?"

Caring for my father ended after six intense weeks, but during that short time, fears haunted me. I was afraid he was in pain. Afraid he would die. Afraid he would live, but as a dialysis-bound invalid. Afraid my mom would collapse. Afraid I would have to make decisions on his care that I didn't want to make. Afraid I'd be in trouble at work because I was staying at the hospital in California. Afraid I'd come unglued myself. And my experience with my dad, relatively short as it was, is a mere shadow of what some caregivers—perhaps *you*—are going through.

When a cold draft of fear blows through you,
Turn to Jesus.
He understands your fear:
Fear that your compassion may break; your strength give out.
He restores your faltering heart.
He revives your loving spirit.
He refreshes you and makes you whole
Your task is difficult and fraught with fear.
But Jesus understands.
Pray for his help
That you may give care
Freely, selflessly and joyfully.
> —A prayer by my friend, caregiver Sally Wunsch

Oh God, from my fear of the unknown,
Deliver me.
From my fear of the future,
Save me.
From my fear of personal weakness,
Liberate me.
> —Barbara Bartocci

FEELING TRAPPED

"I need help," read the message posted on a caregiver's website. "My husband has Parkinson's. He has not been out of the house in a year and a half. I serve his meals in the living room because he gets dizzy-headed when he walks. He's afraid to sit in our dining room chairs for fear he can't get back up. He's afraid to get too far from the bathroom.

"Now I'm afraid, too. Afraid to leave the house for fear something will happen to him. When I do leave, even if it's just to get groceries, he calls my cell phone every few minutes. HELP. What should I do? I feel very, very trapped."

Dear Lord, please bless and guide those of us who are caregivers. It's a fearsome thing to have to shoulder all the care for someone, especially someone who is afraid. May all caregivers everywhere be willing to call for help, and in Thy goodness, grant us an answer that can be heard. Amen.

ACCEPTING

Jodie's widowed dad lives in a care facility that is four states away. "He was active his entire life," she says. "He ran marathons. Loved to hike. Some of my best memories are of the hikes we took together when I was a kid. Last year, though, he had a stroke that paralyzed him. My wonderful, active father had to be placed in a nursing home. It breaks my heart."

Her brother and sister-in-law live nearer and see him more often. But it's too far for Jodie to drive to on a weekend, and airfare is expensive. She tries to make do with phone calls and letters and an on-site visit every four or five months, but she's terribly afraid it's not enough.

Oh God, my mind says, "You're doing all you can," but my heart is burdened and heavy with guilt because I feel I should do more. Some days, worry stays with me like a nagging toothache. Grant me the humility to realize I am not in control of all life's circumstances. Strengthen me to embrace my loved one in daily prayer, even though I'm unable to add a physical embrace. And help me feel compassion, not only for my loved one, but for myself. Amen.

CHANGING ROLES

When I was caring for my mom while she had cancer, there was a moment in the hospital when she looked frightened. No, it was more than that—for an instant, her eyes went *black* with terror as she was told about an upcoming procedure.

No matter how grown-up we are, we never want to see a parent look so terrified. Parents are the ones who took care of us when *we* felt scared. I reached for my mother's hand and murmured, "It's going to be okay, Mom" and gradually, her shoulders relaxed. She closed her eyes. But as our fingers stayed entwined, I understood for the first time how completely our roles had reversed.

Oh Lord, grant me strength in my new role. Help me convey to my loved one the reassuring words of Psalm 91: "You will not fear the terror of the night, or the arrow that flies by day. . . .

Because you have made the Lord your refuge, the Most High your dwelling-place, no evil shall befall you, no scourge come near your tent." Help me remember that I, too, shall find refuge in the Lord, for you are my God and in you I put my trust. Amen.

RENEWAL

The sound of the morning alarm brings a small groan from Allison. She yearns to turn over and sleep for another hour, but staying in bed is not in her schedule, so she flings off the covers.

Twice in the night she had to get up to help her mother to the bathroom. Her mother is unsteady on her feet, and a few weeks ago, when Allison didn't get up right away, her mother fell. "Thank goodness, she didn't break her hip, but she got an awful bruise and it scared us both," said Allison.

When Allison was going through her divorce, it had seemed like a good idea to move in with her mother. She thought it would be an interim stop, but in the two years since she moved in, her mother has grown increasingly frail, so Allison has stayed. It's wearing her down in ways she didn't expect.

Oh Lord, I'm so very tired. Help me to remember that I chose to do this path. I pray in the words of your apostle Paul: "We are hard pressed on every side, but not crushed; perplexed, but not in despair; struck down but not destroyed." Renew me this day as you renewed your servant Paul. Amen.

MONEY FEARS

After their daughter's horrific automobile accident, Marna managed to get six months unpaid leave so she could care for her. Katie, who's sixteen, was a passenger in a car that was hit head on. She faces months of rehabilitation. "Even with insurance, Katie's medical bills are *huge*," said Marna. "I worry all the time about how we're going to pay for it."

Dear Lord, sometimes I, too, get consumed with money worries. My faith has been weakened by my loved one's many needs. Yet your son, Jesus, said, "So do not worry about tomorrow, for tomorrow will bring worries of its own. Today's trouble is enough for today" (Matt 6:34). And in the prayer he gave all of us, we are told to say in confidence, "You give us each day our daily bread." Please help me focus my thoughts on this day only. Strengthen me to let go, and let tomorrow worry about itself. Amen.

NEW REALITY

St. Theresa's is considered a very good nursing home.

Still, every week when Gloria walks inside the cheerful blue and white lobby, what she notices——even more than the silk flowers at the receptionist's desk or the framed seascapes on the wall—is the faint odor of urine. In her mother's room, the walls are hung with family pictures and two crayoned drawings by Gloria's grandchildren. But here, too, she smells the peculiar aroma of old age and sickness, only partially masked by a rose-scented body mist. The woman in the bed is wizened and frail, and bears little resemblance to the lively, active mother Gloria remembers. When Gloria bends to kiss her and murmur, "Mom, it's me," her mother stares at her blankly.

Oh God, it's a fearful thing to see visible signs of deterioration in someone I love. Part of me rebels and wants to run away; another part is horrified to think I might end up the same way. Then I feel ashamed. Help me, Lord, to love and appreciate my loved one as she is right now. Every life contains both light and shadow. Help me to "be not afraid" of the shadows. Amen.

Sometimes, God's grace appears to us through people we encounter. Or events that occur. Or particular words we read or hear at just the right time. And sometimes God asks us to participate. So here are the first "Holy Action" steps to help you when you're coping with caregivers' fears.

QUICK STEPS OF HOLY ACTION

1. Take one small step. Whatever your biggest fear, think of *something* you can do in the next twenty-four hours to lessen it. It doesn't need to be a big step. Something easy like a phone call to a friend, a little on-line research to learn more, a ten-minute walk, or ten minutes of prayer. Doing *something* will help you feel more in control.
2. Breathe. The more fearful we feel, the more likely we are to breathe in short, shallow bursts. Studies have found that deliberate, slow, deep breathing can physically calm you and generate positive chemicals in your brain.

FEAR

3. Relive tranquility. To interrupt fearful thoughts, remember a soothing experience—an early-morning walk on a beach, quiet fishing on a lake, holding your sleeping child—in as much detail as possible. Harvard research has shown that when you mentally relive a carefree time, your body recreates the calming chemicals that were present when you experienced it. You begin to feel less apprehensive and more in control.

4. Challenge your fears. Studies have found that most of the fears people express *do not* come to pass. When you catch yourself in fearful thinking, stop and write down your thought. Look at it objectively. How likely is it to happen? If the worst should happen, what would you do? Think out a plan of action. Write your fears down for one week, and go back and reread the following week. If you see that most of what you feared never happened, it will help you put fearful thoughts into a better perspective.

5. Turn fear into problem solving. Some fears can be restated as problems to solve. For instance, *"I'm afraid I'll lose my own health"* can be restated as *"I need to stay healthy."* Then write down ten possible solutions. Don't stop until you come up with ten, even if some seem absurd.

6. Read aloud the Twenty-third Psalm. in a slow, insightful way. Do it three times a day for one week (maybe at every mealtime). Notice how these ancient words of faith help your mind and soul to feel restored. Notice especially the power of the first line. It states a simple fact:

"The Lord is my shepherd, I shall not want.
    He makes me lie down in green pastures;
he leads me beside still waters;
    he restores my soul.
He leads me in right paths
    for his name's sake.
Even though I walk through the darkest valley,
    I fear no evil;
for you are with me;
    your rod and your staff—
    they comfort me.

You prepare a table before me
    in the presence of my enemies;
you anoint my head with oil;
    my cup overflows.
Surely goodness and mercy shall follow me
    all the days of my life,
and I shall dwell in the house of the Lord my whole
life long."

You might also recite the psalm with plural pronouns ("we"),
    thinking of your loved one at the same time.

7. Schedule your fear: Visualize all your fearful worries
    stuffed into a big bag. Once a day for up to thirty minutes,
    pull them out of the bag. Feel them. Caress them. *Wallow*
    in them. But when thirty minutes are up, stuff them back

into the bag. Tell yourself that tomorrow at the same time you're allowed to pull them out again. This works because you're not asked to totally give up worry, which would probably seem impossible. But by scheduling it, you keep it from overwhelming you. Researchers at Penn State University found that this technique actually reduced worrying by about forty percent among subjects tested. Even if it takes a few days before you're able to truly leave your worry in its bag, I encourage you to keep trying. I've stuffed my own fears into a bag, and I know how that helped!

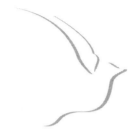

CHAPTER THREE
GRIEF

It's called caregivers' grief: the relentless on-going process brought about, not by a loved one's death, but by the changed aspects of their life, and inevitably, the life of the caregiver.

Riza, whose husband Tod was diagnosed with early-onset Parkinson's disease, told me, "I've accepted the reality of my husband's disease and its day to day impact, but I am still grieving the loss of *my* dreams." She sighed so deeply, I wanted to reach over and hug her. Riza and Tod are in their thirties. Now their plans for children, for the continuation of Tod's career, and for the ordinary activities they enjoy—like hiking and camping in the nearby Colorado mountains—have changed. Of course she laments the change.

Major illness impacts all family members. For some, there's the anticipatory grief of knowing a loved one is terminally ill; for others, like Riza, there is grief as she grapples with the loss of the future she had planned. No matter what we've lost, we need to allow ourselves time to mourn.

You may be thinking, as many caregivers do, "Mourn? Who's got the *time*? I have too much to *do*." Besides, you may add, "Who am I to complain? I don't suffer the physical pain my loved one feels. I'm not the one having medical procedures, or feeling the loss of physical mobility or mental agility. I'm not facing death."

But denying our feelings only sends them deep inside, and that's where they can fester. I've learned that emotions are neither good nor bad; they just *are*. Be honest in acknowledging what you feel. Caregivers' grief seldom comes in a neat, orderly package: you might feel tearful and hopeful at the very same time. Your emotions can take as many twists and turns as your loved one's illness.

A Would-be Runaway's Prayer
Oh Lord, Here is my confession.
A part of me wants to run away.
Wants to leave all of this behind.

The messiness. The turmoil. The tears.
I want to escape to a place that is safe.
Someplace warm and sunny. And happy.
But I remember what the poet Francis Thompson wrote
about God:
"I fled Him, down the nights and down the days;
I fled Him, down the arches of the years;
I fled. . . from those strong Feet that followed,
followed after."
And in Isaiah I read,
"I am your God and will
Guide you in the direction you should journey."
So I stop. I will not flee. I will not run away.
But as I travel this journey
I did not choose, humbly do I pray,
Strengthen me to cope with the messiness.
The turmoil.
And most of all,
Comfort me and my loved one.
Help us to bear our tears.

SMALL LOSSES

We were sitting in a caregiver's circle, a half dozen of us, when I asked, "What are some of the *little* griefs—the small sadnesses—that you think go along with caregiving?" At first, there was silence, and then, tentatively, I heard, "I grieved when Jack got so sick he couldn't do his daily crossword puzzle."

Soon, our voices tumbled over each other.

"Watching Ginny edge her way along with her walker. This is a woman who used to run marathons."

"Hearing Bob repeat himself, saying the same thing over and over."

"I miss time for gardening. It's a real sadness to have no flowers this year."

"Going to movies together, and eating at our favorite Thai restaurant afterwards."

"It grieves me that we don't talk about what's really bothering us. It's like we live in separate cages."

"I'm sad because my wife is so short-tempered with our kids. They don't understand that it's her illness talking."

"Opting out of my forty-year high-school reunion."

"No sex life." (And, amid laughter, this response: "You call that a *little* grief?")

Dear God, Nothing is so trivial in our lives that it goes unnoticed by you. You count the very hairs on our heads. Your son Jesus encouraged us to pray in confidence, not only for what is great and large, but for what is little and concrete. In total assurance I turn, trusting that you know the small sadnesses that are part of my life right now and that your love will help me bear and move beyond them.

SO MANY LITTLE GRIEFS

So many responses emerge when caretakers talk about their "little griefs."

"The first day Evelyn went permanently into her wheelchair."

"When the doctor told Dan he couldn't drink coffee any more. For years, sipping espresso together had been our morning ritual."

"Being forced to keep secrets because my sister didn't want to talk about her condition."

"Though my daughter Lorri went blind, she could still see light until a year ago, when it all went black. She was so angry and depressed! I grieved with her. It's hard when you can't 'make it all well' for your child."

"Bob had such talent for making people laugh. When he was in the early stages of Alzheimers, he tried to tell the same funny stories, but they came out wrong. I *cringed* for him."

"I miss the talkative, interactive, feisty guy I used to live with."

Oh Lord there is so much in caretaking that I cannot control. The only real power I have is the one I've been reluctant to use: the power of surrendering my will to God's. Martin Luther said, "When we lay our need before God in prayer, we must not prescribe to God the measure, manner, time, and place [for response], for God will surely do what is right for us." Very well, oh Lord, take my reluctant surrender and transform it with your grace as I pray, "Thy will be done." Amen.

A DIFFERENT SEASON

Shelly's mom was fiercely independent. But at eighty-eight, she was troubled by age-related macular degeneration which left her legally blind, and an inner ear problem which affected her balance. One day, when Shelly dropped by, she found her mother on her kitchen floor, unconscious. She had fallen and hit her head. Shelly knew her mom could no longer live alone, but it wasn't easy, persuading her to move into an assisted living facility. She protested all the way, and the more she protested, the guiltier and more conflicted Shelly felt.

Oh Lord, moving into a nursing home is very hard. My loved one grieves the loss of independence, and I'm being blamed. There is a lot of anger when I visit. I have searched my soul, but cannot find another answer. Help me listen with patient understanding, and grant us each the willingness to accept these new circumstances. Sweeten my loved one's bitter heart as we acknowledge the truth of Ecclesiastes: To everything a season. Amen.

QUICK STEPS OF HOLY ACTION

1. Give yourself time. When we're thrown into unexpected, unasked-for change, it takes a while to accept it. Don't be in too big a hurry. It's important to work *through* your grief, not try to deny or go around it. Working through takes time.

2. Ride your pain. Women who give birth learn to pant and "ride the pain" much as a surfer rides a wave. Emotional pain is no different. Feel it, go into it, and ride it out.

It *will* lessen, and you will have a respite before the next "wave" comes. Gradually, the periods of rest will grow longer. Trust the process.

3. Find support. Support groups exist for almost every kind of caregiver. People who have walked in your shoes will know best what to say and what guidance to offer. No one should try to go it alone. At the end of this book, you'll find resources to help you.

4. Pray daily. So much is outside of your control that it's important to remind yourself—through daily prayer—that your loved one ultimately is in God's hands. You may think you don't have time for prayer. The truth is, you can't afford *not* to take time.

5. Don't be dismayed if grief reappears. Your initial care-givers' grief may have subsided when suddenly something will trigger it afresh. "Hearts heal faster from surgery than from loss," wrote columnist Ellen Goodman. It's okay to cry—again—for your loved one or for yourself.

6. Focus on today's "next thing." When you discover yourself slipping into "if only" or "I can't bear it" thoughts, force your mind to focus on today: what is the very next thing you need to do? Then do it.

7. Give up guilt. Don't let guilt add to your stress. You are doing the very best you can. If you regret something you said or failed to do, express your regret, and then move on.

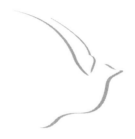

CHAPTER FOUR
HOPE

The quality of hope is so necessary: for our loved ones, and for us as caregivers. To me, a beautiful image is the one in Emily Dickinson's poem:

Hope is the thing with feathers
That perches in the soul,
And sings the tune without the words,
And never stops at all, . . .[1]

Oh Lord, may all caregivers everywhere feel hope's warm flutter amid the burdens of caring for another. Let hope sing in our souls and fly in the face of illness and adversity. Strengthen us, your faithful servants, so that—no matter how heavy the storm—we will always cling, in your name, to our hope.

HUMMING OUR HOPE

When I was caring for my mother, every day I woke up hoping. "I *hope* Mom was able to sleep last night." "I *hope* her pain is less." "I *hope* the MRI will show the cancer hasn't spread." "I *hope* I can reach the doctor today."

At times, my hopes were dashed.

It's one of the hardest things about caregiving, isn't it? The way we grab hold of hope, only to have it sometimes pulled from our fingers.

Hope means to keep living
Amid desperation,
And to keep humming
Even in the darkness.
    —Barbara Bartocci

My friend Sandy who was at the side of her husband Ray in his desperate two-year battle against renal cancer, said "So many days, that's what it came down to: Despite the darkness and desperation, a choice to stay hopeful and keep humming."

Dear God, humbly do I pray: help me choose to stay hopeful. Help me hum in the darkness today. Amen.

Hoping is knowing that there is love.
It is trusting in tomorrow.
It is falling asleep
And waking again
When the sun rises.
In the midst of a gale at sea,
It is discovering land.
In the eyes of another
It is finding compassion.
As long as there is still hope
There will also be prayer.
and God will be holding you
In his hands.[2]

A CAREGIVER'S FORMULA

Jeanne cares for her husband Jake, who has metastasized liver cancer, and she follows the hopeful PCL formula: You Pray, you Cry, you Laugh.

She explained, "Jake and I start each day by praying together. We pray to find the strength we need for that day. And we hopefully affirm what the Lord's Prayer promises: that the Father will give us *this day* our daily bread—not just bread for our bodies, but nourishment for our souls.

"Mostly, we try and skip the Cry part and go directly into Laughter because laughter can trigger the immune system in a positive way. So we talk about the fun we've had and how much we'll enjoy life when Jake is well again. We play cards and put together jigsaw puzzles. We watch DVD movies—funny movies! And I clip cartoons that I think will make Jake smile."

"Even when we do cry—and I admit, there are days when we do —we look for something to laugh about later." Jeanne lifts her hands. "Really, what else can you do?"

Oh Lord, I, too, commit to starting each day with prayer. If my loved one feels uncomfortable praying out loud with me, I will say a silent prayer. And I will consciously look for the comical in each day, for surely hope and laughter go hand in hand. Let me affirm that "I am cheerful and have a great sense of humor." When I do cry, scatter my tears among peals of laughter as hopeful medicine to restore the soul. Amen.

SOMEDAY A CURE

"Hoping for a cure is what keeps us going," says Monica, whose fourteen-year-old daughter, Angie, was diagnosed with cystic fibrosis at age ten. Monica never dreamed that she and her husband, Larry, might each carry the flawed gene that produces CF. Their hopes are pinned on gene therapy. Someday, scientists may learn how to insert a normal gene into CF cells to replace a defective one. They hope this treatment will come during Angie's lifetime. Meanwhile, Angie takes her medications, spends time in the hospital, and, every day, lets her mother pound her chest for an hour to shake loose the web of deadly mucus in her lungs.

Oh God, some miracles happen through the imagination and power of our incredible brains. I give thanks for the many discoveries of human minds, and I ask a special blessing on all research scientists who seek cures to chronic and deadly diseases. Help me tap into my imagination and hold on to my hope as I think of ways to help my loved one today. Amen.

WHEN HOPES DIFFER

Karen wanted her husband, Don, to get a bone marrow transplant. She hoped it might stave off a return of his T-cell lymphoma. But after a rough bout with chemo, his cancer had gone into remission, and Don was finally feeling good again. He didn't want to go through the year-long rigors of a transplant with all its potential side effects.

"Look," said Don, "I'm seventy-four. Even if the transplant doesn't kill me—which it could, you heard the doctors— I'll feel rotten for a year. And there's still no guarantee the lymphoma won't come back. I've had a good run, and I'd rather enjoy whatever life I have left. Play with the grandkids. Go fishing at the lake." He wrapped an arm around Karen. "Spend time with you."

Tears pooled in Karen's eyes as she described the scene. Despite her entreaties, Don was adamant. He didn't want a transplant.

Oh Lord, there are times when I would make a different choice for my loved one. Help me align my hopes with his, and to remember that I am not the patient. As much as I might think

I know what's best, it's not my body. Or my pain. Or my life. Give me the strength to let go and honor the choices my loved one makes. Help me remember that You are ever present, and we can trust in your goodness, whatever turn our lives take. Amen.

FROM BITTERNESS TO HOPE

I see Jane almost every Sunday, pushing her son's wheel-chair down the church aisle for Holy Communion. Her son is a beautiful boy of ten with dark curly hair, but his arms jerk uncontrollably from cerebral palsy. When I learned that she has a second disabled son, and that her husband had left her, I wondered how she managed.

One day we talked, and she admitted that for a long while, she had felt very bitter. "After George left, I *really* shook my fist at God." A turn-around began when an older couple from church, the Thomases, offered to drive Jane and her sons to Sunday services. Soon, they were helping her in other ways. "It was like being adopted by two loving grandparents," said Jane. In the face of such love—and their active assistance with her sons—Jane's bitterness began to dissipate. Today, she has renewed her hope in life's goodness.

Oh Lord, Scripture warns against letting a bitter root cause trouble (Hebrews 12:15). Instead, let me heed the words of the living Christ, "Trust strongly in me and have perfect hope in my Love and Mercy."[3] Help me see when Christ's mercy appears in my life through the actions of others. Amen.

LIFE'S MYSTERY

"My husband had five chronic, degenerative conditions, including osteoporosis, Parkinson's, and pulmonary fibrosis," said Mary, a pretty woman who looks younger than her seventy years. She shook her head as if hardly able to believe it, even now. "For more than twenty years I watched his health decline and his pain increase. His vertebrae were crumbling. He needed oxygen. All during those years, I prayed, often desperately, sometimes despairingly: "Oh God, please help ease his pain. Help me to bear it too. Take away my anger and his fear. Give us both hope and strength."

Mary says she found hope and comfort in repeating these words from the first song of Isaiah (12:2):

Surely God is my salvation;
I will trust, and will not be afraid,
for the Lord God is my strength and my might;
he has become my salvation.

Dear Lord, your will for us is not pain, yet pain stalks my loved one relentlessly. Give me courage to embrace these words: "In the prayer of hope, no guarantees are asked, no conditions posed, and no proofs demanded, only that we expect everything from the Sacred Other without binding him in any way. Hope is based on the premise that the Other gives only what is good." Please help my loved one and me find what is good in this pain-filled place. Amen.

HOPE FOR A GOOD DEATH.

When my friend Jennifer lay in the hospital's palliative care wing, dying of lung cancer, her room became a soft-lit oasis of serenity. She requested a harpist to play in her room, and this was arranged. A close friend brought a kitten to lie in bed with her. Although it was difficult for Jen to breathe, she asked not to be over-sedated, because she wanted to plan her funeral—the hymns and Scripture readings that meant the most to her. And she wanted to interact with family members who were coming.

Her friend and physician, Dr. Richard Sosinski, wrote this paragraph about Jen's final hours: "The last night that she was responsive, a beautiful sunset was visible through the window. While alone with her, I told her that I thought the end was very near. She asked, 'You mean I'm just going to slip away?' 'Yes,' I said, 'Quietly slip away.' She asked for her sister to sit by her side, and for the others that were there to sit quietly in her room. Just before I left, she voiced her final words to me, 'Keep in touch.'" Jen died a few hours later.

Oh Lord, the transition we call death is but a natural part of God's plan, a journey from one state of being to another. Scripture says, "For God so loved the world, that he gave his only Son, that whoever believes in him shall not perish but have eternal life." And Jesus said, "Do not let your hearts be troubled. Believe in God, believe also in me. In my Father's house there are many dwelling-places. If it were not so, would I have told you that I go to prepare a place for you?" (John 14:1–2). What hope is in that promise! Grant me the grace, when it is time, to help my loved one's transition be one of peace, serenity, and hope. Amen.

QUICK STEPS OF HOLY ACTION

1. Surround yourself with hopeful people. A friend of mine, while going through chemotherapy, was visited several times by a neighbor whose wife had died of cancer. He was so doleful that my friend finally said, "I appreciate your coming to visit, but if you can't be more cheerful, I'd rather you not come." She knew she needed to be with people who had a positive frame of mind. She was right, for studies show that people generally reflect the attitude of those around them.

2. Affirm the value of each day. Poet Robert Frost said, "In three words I can sum up everything I've learned about life. It goes on!" Let this be a daily prayer, said aloud: "Life goes on!" Dedicate yourself to making the most of each day, whatever your circumstances, and don't flounder in yearnings for what "might have been."

3. Build hope around the possible. What is something to hope for today that could actually happen? Your loved one has more appetite? You're able to find time to take a walk? The MRI shows good news? If you act as if something hopeful is going to happen, you may discover it does. Just keep your hopes in the realm of possibility.

4. Hope for healing, not a cure. The word "healing" comes from the Anglo-Saxon word *haelen*, meaning to "make whole." When you pray for healing, you are praying for wholeness, and not only for your loved one, but for yourself. If a physical cure is not possible, you can still hope for the consolation of a peaceful end in which your loved one has come to terms with life and feels ready to go on. And you can ask yourself, "What will help *me* feel more whole?" (A good question to write about in your journal.)

5. Keep a journal. A journal is less about what is happening in your life and more about your responses to what's happening. Writing is a good way to process our feelings during stressful times, and—as one caregiver said— "writing in a journal is a lot cheaper than a shrink." I use hard-cover, blank-page books, the kind you find in bookstores.

6. Join other advocates. A dozen caregiver-advocacy groups have sprung up in recent years, pushing for legislation and giving hope by dispensing information. Parents of special needs children, especially, have been fervent advocates and their persistence has paid off in educational opportunities, research funding, and adult housing options for their children. The Internet will help you locate the associations and advocacy groups that are best for you. Consider becoming an advocate, remembering the phrase, "God helps those who help themselves."

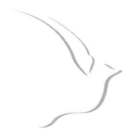

CHAPTER FIVE
CHALLENGES

I've wondered if care-giving is harder than we expect because we don't know *what* to expect. Who *plans* to become a care-giver? Who *plans* to need care? All our expectations are on staying healthy. We want our parents to stay independent and mobile. We want to deliver healthy babies. And who thinks, on their wedding day, that an active spouse might acquire a debilitating disease? So the challenges that come with caregiving catch us unaware and unprepared.

The Kaleidoscope Prayer
Beloved Lord,
My life has shifted,
Like a kaleidoscope turning.
My view of the future
Has been altered.
I did not ask for this change.
I was comfortable with my life as it was.
Yet I trust in your loving concern
To strengthen me.
And while the kaleidoscope may have turned.
Help me see that the new design—though different—
Can still be beautiful.
    —Barbara Bartocci

Lord, remind me, please, that one of your gifts is time.
When it feels like so much is happening all at once,
I need to remember to take one thing at a time.
Could you please let me have a little more of your
patience? Patience with the way things are.
Patience with my loved one. And most of all,
patience with myself.
Lord, I know you have all the time in the world.
Remind me to rest patiently
In your timeless love.
    —Barbara Loots, my friend and a caregiver

HANGING ON TO THE ROLLER COASTER

"It's been a roller coaster," said my friend Lois. Two weeks earlier, her husband Wayne, an avid golfer and tennis player, had gone to the doctor because of fatigue and a fever that wouldn't go away. He was sent to the hospital. After several days of testing, doctors diagnosed Wayne with a terminal liver disease. Before Lois had a chance to contact Hospice, more tests brought a new diagnosis: Wayne was very ill but not terminal. She could take her husband home.

He is still at home, slowly recuperating with the aid of visits from a home nurse and a physical therapist. Lois took leave from her job to stay with him. "I'm incredibly grateful that Wayne is still with me, but I'm reeling. Everything happened so suddenly. So fast. He went from perfectly healthy to nearly dead to slowly recovering. All in just two weeks! It's hard to wrap my mind around it."

That's what can happen in the acute phase of care-giving: adrenaline jerks you up, then down, then up and down again.

Jesus, when your disciples feared their fishing boat might capsize in the rolling waves, they called to you for help. I, too, call on you. Help me hang on. Keep me from tipping over. Most of all, give my loved one and me the strength for a ride we never expected to take.

FINDING SMALL GIFTS

Claire's eighty-eight-year-old mother has lived with them

for the past two years, ever since Claire's dad died. "Jim is terrific," says Claire, referring to her husband. "He's got a great sense of humor and he knows how to make us laugh. But it's still very wearing." Her mother has rheumatoid arthritis and spends most of her time in a wheelchair. Their house isn't built for the disabled, which creates logistical problems, and Claire had to quit her job, which adds financial pressure.

"Mom says, 'I don't want to be a burden,' and I tell her, 'You're not.' I know that living with us has extended her life, and I'm glad about that, but. . . . . . ." A pause. A sigh. "It is harder than I thought it would be."

Please aid me in sorting my confused feelings, oh Lord. Maybe the question I need to ask is not "Why?" but "What?" What is there to learn in this particular vineyard? God knows I didn't choose it, and when I start comparing my life to those of my friends who don't have my burdens, it's easy to fall into self-pity. Help me refocus, dear God. Help me to look at just this day, and find the good in it. Help me feel gratitude for small things. And most of all, if just for today, grant me the gift of laughter. Amen.

STAYING WITH A FRIEND

When my friend Sally started chemotherapy, I offered to stay with her for the first week. Sally lived alone; she was frightened. "I'll bring my laptop," I said. "I can work at your house just as easily as I can at my own."

Her medical regimen was difficult. She developed mouth

sores. She had no appetite. I spent time in her kitchen experimenting with different foods that might seem palatable. She needed help to go to the bathroom. She couldn't get warm. As I brought her another blanket, I realized it was very troubling to me to see my friend in such distress.

But here's what truly dismayed me. I felt awkward in her house. Her kitchen was unfamiliar. I didn't sleep well in her guest room. It was hard to be away from my own routines. Finally, I had to acknowledge that moving into the home of someone who is gravely ill is a lot harder than I had thought it would be.

Beloved Lord, I am grateful for the opportunity to be a help to my friend even though it hasn't been easy. Prayerfully, I recall the words of your son, Jesus: Truly I tell you, just as you did it to one of the least of these who are members of my family, you did it to me" (Matt 25:40). May these words strengthen my resolve and compassion. And next time I will be more realistic in my expectations. Amen.

PATIENCE

"My mom takes eleven medications," reports Irene, "and sometimes she forgot to take one or two. So I made a paper chart, copied it thirty-one times, one for each day of the month, and told her to check off each medicine as she took it. Then I began dropping by two or three times a week just to double check on her meds. And I discovered that sometimes she skipped a medication. *Deliberately.* She said she gets tired of taking so many. And some of the capsules are so big they choke her. It's very frustrating to me. Doesn't she realize she can't keep living independently if she doesn't take her meds?"

Oh Lord, when my caregiving efforts are ignored, I get snappish and angry. But love is both patient and kind (1 Cor 13:4). So I pray for patience—especially the patience to listen and to respond to my loved one's concerns. And when I've gone as far as I can go, help me accept that now may be the time to involve someone else to share in the chores of caregiving. Amen.

LONELY

Some might think June is a lucky caregiver. Although her eleven-year-old daughter, Rachel, was born severely afflicted with Down syndrome and related physical problems, their state's Medicaid program authorizes a personal care attendant for twenty-five hours a week, plus a behavior specialist who comes five hours a week to supplement June's home schooling of her daughter.

So June has some help. But it's hard to keep attendants because pay is low, and her daughter expresses such heartache every time an attendant leaves that, sometimes, says June, she wonders if it's worth it to rehire. "Yet I need the help because I'm the one in the family who shoulders the responsibility. My husband's way of dealing with Rachel's problems is to avoid talking about them. It leaves me feeling very lonely."

Oh Lord, I, too, feel lonely. None of my close friends or family have walked this way, and I see their impatience when I try to talk about my caregiving problems. The Gospel of Matthew says that Jesus often went off by himself to a "lonely place" to pray, but in my lonely place, prayer seems leaden, meaningless. I long for someone who understands. Where, oh Lord, must I look to find it? Help me to figure out an answer. Amen.

EMBARRASSED

Since his stroke, Patti has had to help her eighty-year-old dad with private matters like using the toilet. "He's mortified," she says, "and I'm embarrassed. Neither one of us knows how to handle it."

Lord, help me remember that if humans are made in the image of God, then everything about our bodies is sacred, including our most intimate functions. Through the power of your Holy Spirit, give me the right words to help my loved one realize there is no shame in accepting my help. Amen.

GIVING CHOICES

Jean's widowed mother was fiercely determined to remain independent, and as long as Jean stopped by two or three times a week, she was able to continue living in her own home. But her eyesight was failing and she'd become forgetful. Sometimes she wore the same blue housedress, with jelly stains on the front, for days at a time. Though Jean brought groceries and even prepared some meals, her mom was likely to shove the dish aside and make a face. "I don't like that. Take it away."

You can tell a child what to do and add, "Because I said so, that's why." But it doesn't always work with elderly parents. When Jean insisted, "Mom, you need to eat more," or, "Mom, put on a clean robe. That one's dirty," her mother would argue, "There's nothing wrong with what I'm wearing." Or, petulantly, "I'll eat what I feel like." It seemed to Jean as if she and her mother argued more and more.

Dear God, give me the empathy to realize how hard it is go from being independent to having other people tell you what you can or cannot do. Give me the wisdom to offer choices. Remind me to allow my loved one to make decisions, large and small, for as long as possible. Amen.

I CAN'T DO THIS

My mother's colon cancer had progressed to the point that a feeding tube had to be inserted directly into her stomach. It needed daily cleaning—with cranberry juice!—and I was warned to keep my hands very sterile when I worked with it. It felt so peculiar to be standing at my mother's side pumping cranberry juice into her stomach. The activity itself wasn't "difficult"—any more than the tube was painful for my mom. But we were both uncomfortable, she that she needed to be fed this way and I that I had to learn to perform such an invasive procedure on my mother.

Oh Lord, in my caretaking duties, I am being asked to do

something that is difficult for me. It is a cross to bear. I used to be so afraid of crosses. Whenever I read the scriptural words, ". . . take up your cross daily and follow me. . . " my response was "No! I don't want to!" But crosses inevitably appear in our lives. So now, prayerfully, the words I count on are these, "Take my yoke upon you and learn from me. . . .for my yoke is easy and my burden is light"(Matt 11:29). Amen.

QUICK STEPS OF HOLY ACTION

1. Don't do it all. Allow the one you care for to do as much for him-or herself as possible. Let your elderly mother clean as much of her own home as she can. Let your spouse continue to write checks and pay bills even if it takes a little longer. People appreciate feeling independent.

2. Involve family members. Don't assume your family knows when you need help. They may be waiting for you to ask or they may need to be given specific tasks. Grandchildren who feel close to a grandparent may be tickled if you give them an assignment.

3. Notice your behavior. If you're trying *too* hard to always be cheerful with the one you're caring for, you may take out your sadness or frustration on other members of your family. If it happens, take a minute to apologize for your irritable—maybe even angry—behavior. Then forgive yourself. Caregiving is one of the most challenging jobs there is—and no one is perfect at it all the time.

4. Avoid guilt trips. Don't feel guilty because you're healthy

and your loved one is not. Instead, give thanks to God for your good health. Each of us has a particular life stream, and we're not called on to become ill because another person is ill. Remember that your good health allows you to offer care to the one you love.

5. Keep your hands busy. Especially if you're spending long, anxious hours at a hospital, consider learning how to crochet or knit. A friend said about knitting, which she took up after her daughter became ill, "It allowed me to start over again, which was very comforting. In my life, I had to keep moving forward, no matter how messy or difficult it became." Keeping your hands and fingers busy is a prayer meditation of its own.

6. Create community with your computer. Whether it's yours or a friend's, a computer can be a useful tool. You can "Google" medical information online. And because many websites have caregiver support groups, consider joining an online community to help you meet your daily challenges. www.caregivingtoday.com is one of the best.

7. Trust your intuition. Intuitive knowledge is a way of knowing without the conscious use of reasoning. It is truly the Spirit within you. You know your loved one better than any medical professional. When treatment options are discussed, if you have a "gut feeling" that it's not workable for *this* patient, speak up. A friend of mine actually stood at her husband's hospital room door, barring the way so the doctor couldn't leave until he listened to her.

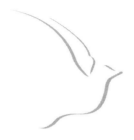

CHAPTER SIX
GIFTS

Recently, I read an anecdote about opera star Beverly Sills. Both of her children were born with disabilities, so there was heartache along the way. Yet Beverly's nickname was "Bubbles." When an interviewer asked her, "How do you manage to stay so happy?" she replied, "Oh, I'm not always happy. But I am always cheerful." She continued, "A happy woman is one who has no cares at all. A cheerful woman is one who has cares but doesn't let them get her down."

The power of that small story has stayed with me.

Happiness is an emotion; cheerfulness is an attitude. Even in the worst of circumstances, I remind myself that I have the power to choose my *attitude*. A cheerful attitude can be a real gift when we're caring for another.

Dear God,
Today instead of the sick room smell,
I give thanks for other aromas.
For coffee beans roasting. And new-mown grass.
For sun-dried bedsheets. And early spring rain.
For chocolate chip cookies, still warm from the oven;
And the rich smell of leather
In a loved one's jacket.
So fragrant! Like incense,
I inhale life's bountiful blessings,
And I breathe my prayer:
Thank You.
  —Barbara Bartocci

Another Prayer of Gratitude
Almighty and Gracious Father,
Behold Your creation.
You made us in Your image.
You gave us our son, our daughter, our father,
Our mother, our spouse, our friend.
With Your help and love, we will keep
Close our memories of

Shared good times
With the one we care for now.
And offer up our difficult days
For the glory of your kingdom.
Blessings are found in all things.
Your Name be praised.
Amen.
    —*Bill Ryan, spiritual director, caregiver, and my friend*

EXTRAORDINARY CHOICES

Some years ago, I interviewed Karen Scates. Karen had agreed to be the legal guardian of Angela, the infant daughter of a teenage mother who belonged to Karen's church. Angela had severe cerebral palsy, triggered by the drug addiction of her birth mother.

By her third birthday, Angela still couldn't sit up, crawl or make intelligible sounds. Friends tried to persuade Karen—who was divorced and had to support herself—to give Angela up. But Karen said, "I look at Angela's sweet, sweet face and feel so much love. Even though she can't speak my name, she *knows* me. I can't give her up."

Like many of Karen's friends, I was amazed that this woman would willingly take on a child with such severe disabilities. But Karen said it was simple: "I love my daughter, and my daughter loves me. And that's enough reward."

Oh Lord, I am awestruck by those who choose the caretaker's path and see love instead of heartache and drudgery.

I did not choose my path, and it sometimes seems overwhelming. Help me walk it willingly. Help me leave behind any resentment, and focus, instead, on the love I feel for the one I care for. Most of all, help me notice all the small ways—the smiles, the hugs, the touch of a hand—in which my love is returned. Amen.

Unexpected Gifts

"We stared at the brown clumps floating in the toilet bowl as if they were jewels, and in a sense they were," said Dottie. For days, her beloved husband had been plagued with diarrhea, an accompaniment to an intestinal infection acquired in the hospital while he was being treated for cancer.

The clumps were good news. It meant the infection might be responding to one of only two drugs that had any chance of healing it. "People don't talk much about bowel movements and fecal matter," said Dottie. "It startled me to realize how important both can be and how eagerly you can examine the contents of a toilet bowl. Before he was diagnosed with cancer, would I ever have thought my husband and I would share such a moment of hopeful euphoria?"

In the name of the Sacred One who became Incarnate, I pray in gratitude. Our bodies are so beautifully designed. So strong. I give thanks for every way in which my own body performs in the way it was intended. I know that in an instant, bodies can become fragile. Let me never take for granted any of our bodies' natural functions. Amen.

AT THE HOSPITAL

"No one really rests in a hospital," says Laurie, whose husband Ted was hospitalized for three weeks. "Every quarter-hour someone is coming in with a thermometer or a needle or to read a chart. And staff changes so often, you don't have a sense of 'your nurse' who knows 'your case.' Instead, you repeat the same information or hear the same questions over and over from different people. And when several doctors are treating different parts of the body, I worry: 'Do they communicate with each another? Does doctor A know what doctor B is prescribing?'"

Dear God, a hospital can be a frightening place, but instead of feeling anxious, help me to appreciate the gift of having a hospital to go to. Help me remember that for those who live in countries of war or poverty—and for some even in this country—a hospital stay is beyond their means. Bless and strengthen those without medical resources. Give me good listening and speaking skills so that I can ask the right questions and hear information correctly, and help me to regard all on the patient-care team as people to value. Amen.

LISTENING

I've been listening to my friend Suz process out loud some of life's new realities. Suz is blonde, petite, and athletic, and never expected to become ill. But six months ago, she was diagnosed with lymphoma. As part of her treatment, she elected to have a bone marrow transplant. "You'll be sick for about a year," doctors warned her.

That's not so bad, Suz thought, I can stand anything for a year.

But complications set in, and Suz has begun to realize: "I can hope to get better, but I'm never going to be exactly the way I was before."

As she tells me this, I wonder how to respond. Should I be cheery and recite hopeful statistics? Should I say, "Buck up, Suz. This is just a rough patch"?

Or should I simply listen? And not say anything?

When her hand touches mine, I know I've made the right choice. "Thank you. It's such a gift to have a friend who doesn't give me a bunch of cheerful platitudes," she says.

Oh Lord, in the words of St. Francis, 'Grant that I may not so much seek to be understood as to understand." Thank you for the gift of grace that enabled me to quietly listen instead of trying to boost my friend's spirits or solve her problem. Grant me always the gift of a listening ear. Amen.

SHARING

Earl and Nancy had such a warm, loving marriage. When Nancy was diagnosed with cancer at the age of fifty-five, Earl was devastated, and during the months when her illness became terminal, he poured his feelings into a journal, part of which he shared with me after Nancy's death.

"Nancy's illness is like a long flight of descending stairs," he wrote. "The steps only go down. You try to stay on each step for a time, until the next step down, but there's never any hope of climbing up, only going down to the end, which seems shadowed and not quite visible.

"I want to ask her: am I doing the right things? Do you have concerns that we haven't discussed? Are you frightened? I know I am. My pain is nothing compared to hers, but it is real and overpowering at times. I hurt so for her, and I feel so helpless."

Dear God, bless those who generously share their feelings with me. They let me know I'm not alone. Connecting with others in a genuine, open way is such a meaningful gift. Give me the grace to open up to others about my experience, especially when I think it will give them a boost. And whenever we share, may your Spirit be there to strengthen all of us. Amen.

PIZZA

Fred was a corporate vice president in his late forties when he was diagnosed with ALS. He and his wife Gwen were devastated because ALS (Lou Gehrig's disease) is a terminal neurological illness that leaves your mind intact but progressively destroys your body. Gwen does not deny their daily difficulties, but she does remember one special night, a few months after Fred's diagnosis, when six close friends stopped by with pizza. "Somehow, that evening, we were able to set aside our awful fears for the future, and just enjoy the talk and laughter and warm feelings," says Gwen. It helped that these same friends continued to reach out in support.

Oh God, thank you for friends who do not fall away. It is a fearsome, lonely time when illness strikes, and just when the need for constancy is greatest, some become frightened and disappear. May a special blessing fall on those who stay. And please, oh Lord, let me not suffer from the pride that makes me think I have to go it alone. Give me the humility and courage to reach out to others for help. Amen.

VISITING DAD

Jenny's dad is in a nursing home. "I've learned there's no point in visiting too early because that's when the aides and sometimes the doctors are making their rounds. So unless I'm trying to reach a doctor, I go by closer to noon. I've arranged with my boss to consider that my lunch hour. My dad and I sit together in the sun room where wide windows sprinkle us with light. I used to bring Dad crossword puzzles—once upon a time, he loved to do them—but now he's content to simply sit. Sometimes, we don't talk at all. I just sit beside him and hold his hand. He likes it when I hold his hand."

Oh Lord, just as my parent once held my hand to keep me safe as I crossed the street, now I give thanks that I can hold my parent's hand as he or she crosses over into a new phase of life. Give us both the courage to face the inevitable changes that age and illness have brought. Help me remember the worth of a loving touch even when I can do nothing else. Amen.

GIFTS

SEEING DIFFERENTLY

A friend sent this e-mail:

"The first time I had lunch with my mother in her assisted living facility, everyone looked the same to me. Old. Wrinkled. Thinning white hair. Humped shoulders. But after a few visits, I began to see individuals: Gloria has Parkinson's so she shakes a little, but she has a wide, generous smile. She used to be a hairdresser and still loves to gossip. Jane speaks in a whispery voice. She lived on a farm and her hobby was quilting. Harry still likes to do jigsaw puzzles, although he says it's hard for him now because his eyesight is so poor. These are not just "old people." They led active lives before coming to Oak Lawn. They have distinctive personalities. So does my mother, who shares the lunch table with Gloria and Jane and Harry."

Oh Lord, bless me with the wisdom to see people as individuals and not merely lump them into categories— whether it's "old people," "teenagers," "African-Americans," "Latinos," or any other generalized label. Help me to remember that there is only one category that all people fall into—that of "God-holder." I pray to see everyone I meet as an individual who holds, like a candle lit within, the spirit of God. Amen.

SURPRISE HELP

"You never know who will be your biggest support," says Diane. She's a pretty woman, though her face shows the stress she's been living with since her husband, Ben, was diagnosed with cancer. "Remember the Golden Rule? 'Do unto others as you would have them do unto you?'" As I nod, Diane leans toward me. "Well, I experienced the reverse. After Ben got so sick, the one person who helped me most was the very person I had *not* helped." Diane looks a little shame-faced as she relates the story. Her friend Gwen had divorced a few years earlier, and ". . . well, neither Ben nor I wanted to get in the middle of a divorce hassle, so we just—let our friendship go."

Diane ran into Gwen again when she was picking up medicine for Ben. By this time, Gwen had remarried. She looked happy and seemed truly glad to see Diane.

"I told her about Ben's illness, and the very next day, she brought a meal to our house. I was so frazzled. Still working. Caring for Ben. Trying to take care of our daughter. Gwen offered to drive Julie to her softball practice."

Now Gwen comes over once or twice a week. She stays with Ben when Diane needs to get out. Drives their daughter to her sports or band practice. "She's been a truer friend to me than I ever was to her. I'm so grateful," says Diane.

Oh Lord, thank you for the unexpected people who give help. Thank you for those who do not wait to be asked. And for those who just "do it" without having to be told. Thank you for the faithful ones who keep coming by. For all these saints-in-training, I say thanks. May I never take any of them for granted. Amen.

LIFE'S LESSON

Susan's mother knew she was dying, and talked openly about it. Her daughter laughs. "She made lists. Ten people she wanted me to call after she died to tell them what an impact they had had in her life. Three hymns to sing at her funeral. She even made a list of women—all long-time friends—that my father should date after she was gone!" Susan's mom spent her final days looking at family photo albums and scrapbooks from her college days, reminiscing aloud about her life, telling her daughter stories that are now precious to Susan. Her mother no longer apologized because Susan had left her own family to be with her. She said simply, "I'm so glad you're here with me." Susan smiles through tears and says, "My mother included me in her life right up to the end. It was an amazing gift."

Oh Lord, thank you for the intimate connection that exists between my loved one and me. Thank you for the laughter and hugs and—yes—even joy that we have found in the precious moments of each day. Grace us with patience and fortitude to accept what lies ahead, and help us to continue to see the gifts that are here for us in our time together. Amen.

QUICK STEPS OF HOLY ACTION

1. Start a prayer network among those in your church congregation who are caregivers. Agree to pray for each other by name every morning. You might also create a group e-mail (through a service such as Yahoo! Groups) so

caregivers can post notes to one another. Research has shown that people who help others are able to handle their own situations better.

2. Laugh more! As far back as the book of Genesis, it is written, "God has brought laughter for me; everyone who hears will laugh with me" (Gen 21:6). Buy humorous books and tapes as well as inspirational books such as this one. Both types will help keep your spirits up. Did you know that a deep belly laugh does as much for your heart as ten minutes of aerobic exercise? It's true. Look for opportunities to laugh.

3. Write your gratitude. Keep a Gratitude Journal. *I lift up my heart in gratitude for (you fill in the blank).* Each day write down *something* you're grateful for. This practice helped me. Here are some of my "thank you" ideas:
   • Indoor plumbing and a hot shower
   • Your own good health
   • Bountiful food
   • A beautiful sunrise
   • Springtime flowers
   • A small gesture of love from the person you're caring for
   • The assistance of others.

4. Make a "Help Wanted" list. List tasks that people can do for you. For instance: *Pick up laundry. Take the car to be serviced. Make a run to the grocery store. Pick up prescriptions. Return library books. Rent a movie.* Keep the list in your wallet, and when someone asks, "What can I do?" let

them choose from your list. Remember, people *want* to help and will be grateful if you give them some specific opportunities.

5. Maintain your routine. Especially if you're a caregiver for the long-term, give yourself the gift of keeping to the routine you're used to as much as you can. Go to work. Do your exercises. Attend church. Get your hair done. Sticking to the ordinary relieves some of the pressure. Ask friends or family to spell you for two hours every week. Check out community resources. Remind yourself that you can't do it all!

6. Appreciate the gift of advance notice. One of my friends has a fervent wish: that her parents will die suddenly and that she will, too. "None of this lingering-illness stuff for me," says Tina. It *isn't* easy to watch a loved one die, but it does offer the opportunity to make plans, to get legal issues in order, and most of all, to say good-bye, to express love, and if necessary, to make amends. Let us remember that the gift of time offers its own reward.

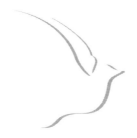

Chapter Seven
Burnout

There may come a moment when you think, "I can't do this any more. I just *can't*." The daily regimen, the interrupted nights, the roller-coaster effect of doctors' diagnoses and counter-diagnoses, or maybe the sheer foreverness with no positive horizon in sight—all threaten to push care-givers into burnout.

Burnout hits when excessive stress makes a person feel hopeless and powerless. Or resentful. Sometimes a caregiver's own health is compromised. One wife was so stressed as she cared for her husband with Alzheimer's that she began showing symptoms of ill health herself. "What if I die before my husband?" she worried.

Feeling isolated is a big component of burnout, so when you're caregiving, it's more important than ever (even if it seems harder) to reach out to friends, relatives, and community support systems.

Here are two prayers for those moments of feeling overwhelmed.

Dear God, I am so angry!
It is too much!
Take this burden from me!
Take it now!
And if you cannot take it,
If it be mine to endure,
Then, oh God, become my partner,
And forge my anger
Into the power I need
To bear the unbearable.
   —*Barbara Bartocci*

Oh God,
Let me not pray to be sheltered from dangers,
But to be fearless in facing them.
Let me not beg for the stilling of my pain,
But for the heart to conquer it. Amen.
   —*Tagore*

TOO MANY PULLS

"Yesterday, my daughter was in a play at her school, my boss asked me to work overtime, and my mother was expecting my visit at her nursing home," said Katherine, her voice shrill and anxious. "I did manage to get to Katie's play, but I had to put off visiting my mom. And as soon as I saw her, I heard the accusation in her voice, 'Why didn't you come yesterday?' Of course, I felt instantly guilty. But also resentful."

Oh Lord, I'm being pulled in too many directions. Sometimes it feels like parts of me are ripping apart. And no matter what choices I make, someone is sure to be disappointed or angry. Please grant me the willingness to be kind to myself and to realize I can only do so much. Help me make wise choices when I have too much on my plate. And then, if I must, help me bear patiently another's disappointment or anger. Amen.

I'M TOO YOUNG!

Kim and Joel were high school sweethearts who married three months before Joel deployed to Iraq with the Marines. After he suffered a TBI—Traumatic Brain Injury—he spent fourteen months in rehabilitation at Walter Reed before returning to his Kansas home town. People injured from TBIs often face lifelong disabilities, not only physically but emotionally. Kim says Joel's personality has changed. "He has trouble concentrating and making decisions, and he can't remember from day to day. Sometimes he totally loses control and his temper seems to be getting worse. This concerns me. I want to stay with him, but it's very, very hard. I'm twenty-three. I didn't expect this."

Dear God, your son, Jesus, said: "Take my yoke upon you and learn from me. . . you will find rest for your souls, for my yoke is easy and my burden is light" (Matt 11:28). But this yoke is not easy and does not feel light. In your mercy, please reshape the yoke to fit my loved one's shrinking shoulders so it does not become too heavy. And because we are yoked together, strengthen me, too. Give me the energy I need to plow this one furrow for this one day. Amen.

POSTPONEMENT

After her divorce, Julie focused on raising her two children. Only when her younger son moved out last year did she start thinking about what *she* might want to do. But before she could depart on her eagerly-planned trip to France, her father was diagnosed with lung cancer.

Julie's an only child, and her mother instinctively turned to her for help. So Julie set aside her travel plans to help care for her dad. Eight weeks after he died, her mother fell down the stairs and broke her hip. Now her mother has moved in with Julie, and Julie no longer talks about travel except as a dream for "sometime, maybe."

I asked Julie, "Do you feel a little trapped? It seems as if you keep doing for others, and never for yourself."

For a moment, she looked wistful. Then she shrugged.

"I love my family." As if that explained it all. And doesn't it? If we love our families, most of us give whatever help is needed even if it means putting our own plans on hold.

Oh Lord, next to you, my family is most important to me. I want to be here for them. But now and then, I daydream. I get impatient with the tug of others' needs and wonder what it might be like to have more freedom. Help me remember why I'm doing what I do. Later, when I am free to pursue my own dreams, I'll get more pleasure from them because I did the right thing when my family needed me. But I confess, oh Lord, sometimes I need your help to remember this. Amen.

Caring for a Lifetime

Marta's younger brother Davy was born with cerebral palsy. "When I was growing up," said Marta, "I watched Davy struggle to talk and heard the garbled way his words came out. I saw his arms wave like windmills because he couldn't control the muscle spasms, and I was so thankful then for my own healthy body. But I had a funny mix of emotions. I understood why my parents focused mostly on Davy, but sometimes I felt just a little resentful.

"Davy and I are both grown now, and my parents have talked to me about my responsibility for Davy's care after they are gone. Of course, I'll do whatever is needed. I love my brother. But though I never talk about it, and feel guilty admitting this, secretly I do sometimes feel as if my whole life has been, well, *burdened* by my brother's illness.

Oh generous Creator, you who know all that we think and feel, even before we might know it ourselves, take my confession of burden and help me see it for what it is—an honest complaint that is only part of what I feel. Larger than my own "dark feeling" of being weighed down, I have another honest feeling of love. When it's my turn to take responsibility, guide me in asking for the support and aid that I, too, will need. Amen.

SIBLING PROBLEMS

"I am *furious* at my brother!" Laurie writes on the message board of a web site for caregivers. "He claims his job keeps him 'too busy' to help take care of Dad, and besides, he lives too far away. But what about *my* job? And my family? I have a terrible time juggling work and kids and helping our dad. At the very least, Ed could take some vacation time and give me a break. But no, he's always got some excuse. He makes me so angry!"

Judging by the sympathetic responses to her outburst, Laurie is not the only sibling who feels put upon. In most families, the adult child who lives closest to elderly parents bears the brunt of their care. If a brother and sister live in the same vicinity, the sister is most often the "hands on" caregiver. Over time, resentments build.

Dear God, it's true. I am seething with resentment because I feel as if the other members of my family are not doing their fair share. I'm tired of always being the one in charge. Yet I can't bring myself to just walk away. I want to do something; I'm just tired of doing it all.

Oh Lord, guide me in doing what I can, and strengthen me to say what I'm no longer able to do. And please, help me to find in my heart forgiveness for my siblings. Amen.

MORE THAN A TRIPLE DOSE

It was an extraordinary set of circumstances. Not long after Shirley's father was diagnosed with early-stage Alzheimer's, her brother, forty-five, suffered a major heart attack. Then her sister's husband learned he had cancer. Six weeks later, the day before Christmas Eve, her mother had a heart attack. Christmas was forgotten as Shirley drove four hundred miles to be with her stricken parents.

Her mother recovered sooner than Shirley's brother, but her dad began wandering off. Concerned for his safety, Shirley moved him to a nursing home. For the next few months, she made frequent visits so her ninety-year-old mother could live independently. But that changed when Shirley's own husband suffered a stroke. "I couldn't keep driving out to see Mom and take care of Harold, too. I had to move Mom into the nursing home. She was so angry! She didn't want to go!"

Happily, her mother did settle in, and Shirley found some relief. But it was short-lived. Her father had grown increasingly violent; she was asked to find him another placement.

"Can you imagine *anything* else happening?" said Shirley, with a shake of her head. "Well, it did. I was diagnosed with breast cancer and my son got a divorce."

Burnout doesn't begin to express Shirley's emotional overload. What saved her, she says, was a church support group. "All of us were going through major life upheavals, but we decided to call ourselves 'Celebrators' because even with all our problems, we wanted to show that life is worth celebrating."

Dear God, heed my prayer, the same prayer Shirley said, over and over: "Give me strength." When so many afflictions come at once, I feel like Job. Grace me with a faith so strong that even in the face of my present difficulties, I, too, will continue to celebrate life. Amen.

A Prayer of Celebration
Oh sovereign God, in your bountiful creation,
Rain falls on the just and the unjust,
Signifying life's Infinite Mystery.
I cannot know your ways; there is much I will never understand.
Yet still, I bow in humble worship
To a power greater than my own.
And even in the darkness,
I choose to live faithfully and to celebrate life.
Hear me oh Lord, and be with me,
Now and forever, Amen.
    —*Barbara Bartocci*

QUICK STEPS OF HOLY ACTION

1. Don't buy into half-truths.

   • Husbands feel that as men they must be strong and take total charge.

   • Women believe that because they promised to love "in sickness and in health," they must always be the sole caregivers if their husbands become ill.

   • Younger women act like superwomen and try to do it all.

   • Daughters may think it's their duty as females and brothers—because they're male—can't be asked to give hands-on care.

   • All family members may take for granted that the person living closest to the one in need automatically becomes the caregiver.

   • Every one of these beliefs is only partially true. Caregiving responsibilities need to be frankly discussed among all parties concerned. It's a good idea, as your parents grow older, to hold this conversation before anyone needs full-time care.

2. Ask for "small bits." It's hard for most of us to ask for help. You may feel more comfortable if you ask for little bits of aid from many people. Ask four people to do one errand each rather than ask one person to do four errands. Ask three friends to take turns picking up your children at school for a week. It helps, too, to think about what

others can realistically deliver. Don't ask a friend to drive fifteen miles to mow your lawn. Turn to a neighbor. When possible, fit your need to the other person's capabilities.

3. Set boundaries. One wife I talked to went home from the hospital every night even though she could have slept in the patient's room. She knew she needed time by herself to recharge *her* batteries. Be realistic about how much you can or cannot do and don't feel guilty about setting limits. When my critically ill father was in the ICU, it was hard to leave him, but I had a work project to finish, so I did fly home for five days. I left my mobile phone number in case my dad's situation worsened.

4. When you are away from the sick room, do your best to think about other things. Try to find something to laugh about!

5. Be alert to depression or Generalized Anxiety Disorder (GAD). Clinical depression is as different from ordinary stress as colon cancer is different from an upset stomach. Learn the symptoms so you can spot them in yourself. GAD shows up as excessive worry; an unrealistic view of problems; restlessness, irritability, or a feeling of being "on edge," and is fairly common among caregivers, especially in acute situations. Anxiety disorder is not the same as depression, but both can be relieved with medication. Cognitive (talking) therapy also helps. The right meds can make a remarkable difference in a

caregiver's outlook. Remember, taking medication doesn't have to be for the rest of your life.

6. Pray your three daily gratitudes. As the last thing before going to sleep, my friend Nora Ellen mentally looks back over her day and acknowledges three things that were helpful. They can be small: "It snowed today." Or, "It *didn't* snow." Or, sometimes, simply: "I made it through the day." She gives thanks for all three. It's a beautiful prayer habit. I began doing it, too. Won't you?

7. Brainstorm. If you're headed for burnout, and your siblings won't or can't help you, can other relatives lend a hand? Can you arrange for senior day care? Are funds available for at-home care, at least part-time? Ask for ideas from others in your situation. Or write the key word that describes your problem in the middle of a piece of paper, and as fast as you can jot down ideas, circling your key word.

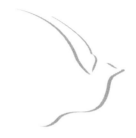

CHAPTER EIGHT
BALANCE

"It's like dancing on a tight-rope while you're juggling a dozen eggs," is the way one care giver described her experience. She was always afraid that—splat!—she would drop one of the eggs and it would break.

Or she would.

How do you stay balanced when you have to add the needs of an ailing or an aged loved one into an already busy life?

When I taught time management seminars, I counseled

my business audiences to set clear priorities. The question to ask is not what you *think* your priorities should be, but what you *want* them to be. While it may not be possible for you to go much beyond "this day" or "this week" in your caregiving, the principle is a useful one.

Take a few minutes to ask yourself prayerfully: "If *my* life as a caregiver could focus on one thing and one thing only, what would that be?" If you added a second thing, what would that be? A third? A fourth? A fifth?

Nancy Lee, a caregiver whose mother is in a nursing home listed:

1. Husband and children
2. Job
3. Exercise
4. Mom
5. Church.

"I'm ashamed of myself," she said, holding up her list. "How can exercise be more important than my mother . . . or going to church?"

But we don't judge our priorities. We simply acknowledge them. Nancy Lee didn't have a close relationship with her mother, so visiting Mom was further down on her list of "wants." She missed exercising, which she'd given up because she felt obligated to her mother. Worse, she felt resentful.

After making her list, she decided to visit her mother for

an hour three times a week instead of five, and on alternate days, use the same hour for exercise, which helped her feel less stressed and better able to cope with her family's needs. She also gave up serving on church committees, acknowledging to herself that "Church is not the same thing as God" and for now, her attendance had to be limited to Sunday service. By acknowledging priorities, she was able to set down one of her eggs instead of simply dropping it and watching it break.

It's not easy. Priorities can't always be followed in such an uncluttered way, especially if your loved one is in a critical situation. But for the long pull, recognizing priorities does help us to make more balanced choices.

Oh Holy One, Scripture says, "But strive first for the kingdom of God and his righteousness, and all these things will be given to you as well"(Matt 6:33). Therefore, before anything else, I pray to experience your presence within. Then keep my steps steady and my spirits high as I figure out daily priorities. Set me free from misplaced guilt as I choose to live in a more balanced way. With your living presence within, I know I am accepted in all that I do because you know I am doing the very best I can. Amen.

MORNING RUN

One of the things I missed most when I began caring for my mother in California was my morning run. Then my mom's sister came for a week. The first morning she was there, I got up early and slipped out of the house. The air was still cool. I heard bird calls, and a dog's bark; the hum of an engine as someone drove off to work. As I crested a hill, I could see across the canyon to the scrubby mesa on the other side. The sky was still tinged with streaks of sunrise and in the distance, I spied a hawk, its wings outspread, catching the wind. I took a deep breath and murmured out loud, "Thank you, God." For that moment, I felt balanced and at one with the world; a world that was larger than my mother's sick room.

After that, I got up early every morning—even after my aunt left—and jogged up the hill behind my parents' house. My mother was sick, yes—terminally so—but she wasn't in danger if I left her alone for thirty minutes. And my morning run not only helped my body, I realized; it helped my soul, giving me stamina for the day ahead.

Dear Lord, thank you for morning minutes. Even though I lose a little sleep, I have some precious time alone to pray or read or walk around the block. It helps me feel more balanced for the rest of the day. Thanks be to God for morning minutes. It is beyond my power to change the big picture, but I can change the small details of life by adopting a cheerful attitude and by the many little ways in which I make my loved one more comfortable. What this means day to day is a willingness to surrender my will. Amen.

Workplace Reprieve

When Pat's husband, Fred, was diagnosed with early-stage Alzheimer's, she was frantic. "I'm still working and love my job," said the sixties-something school administrator, "but Fred couldn't be left alone any longer." Then Pat discovered a nearby center that offered day services for people with Alzheimer's. "Some working parents spend most of their paycheck on their children's day care. I do the same for adult-care. But I thank God for it. At home, our lives are built around Fred's illness. Going to work lets me live my own life again, at least for eight hours."

Dear God, can I ask a friend or relative to come by regularly while I get out for a few hours? Can I be more relaxed about housekeeping? Or ask my kids for more help around the house? If I'm managing financial matters for my loved one, can I let another family member take over? Inspire me with creative wisdom to find a little time to live my own life again. Help me realize in my heart that involving others is not an imposition but an opportunity. Amen.

GOD ALONE

As a 24/7 spousal caregiver, Bill leans on the power of prayer to help him stay balanced. "At this point in the progression of my wife, Carol's, post-polio syndrome, I feel as if my whole *life* is a prayer. I pray for Carol's well-being. I pray that she will have a day free of fatigue and pain. I pray that I will be a good caregiver. I pray that I'll maintain my own personal health." Bill finds a special comfort in this reflection by Teresa of Avila, the sixteenth-century Catholic saint:

Let nothing disturb you
Nothing cause you fear
All things pass. . . .
Whoever has God
Needs nothing else
God alone suffices.[6]

Oh holy Spirit, inspire me with Teresa's unquenchable faith.
Grant me her calm assurance that God alone is sufficient to our
needs. Though our lives are unfolding in a way never planned,
I know we are daily embraced by the Compassionate One.
In faith I affirm that I and my loved one can rest easy in you.
Amen.

WALKING A SACRED CIRCLE

Jenny is a caregiver for her daughter, who has MS and is wheelchair-bound. A chance article on the Internet led her to a nearby church to walk its outdoor labyrinth.

A labyrinth is a path of concentric circles designed to create a centered sense of peace. The design dates as far back as 4500 B.C. One of the most famous is in the floor of the great cathedral in Chartres, France. Unlike mazes, labyrinths have no dead ends. The circular path leads unerringly to the center, and represents our journey through time and experience to God.

"There is so much I *can't* do for my daughter. I have to continually remind myself to just let go and let God," she said. Walking the sacred circle of the labyrinth helped. As she walked, she meditated on God's purpose in her life, and let the labyrinth remind her that at the center of all is God.

Oh Lord, sometimes I feel as if I'm going around in circles, getting nowhere, and with nowhere to go. I pray to mentally enter the sacred space of a labyrinth. May it help me regain my sense of balance and remind me that with God—the Alpha and Omega—there are no dead ends. And no way I can be lost. Amen.

QUICK STEPS OF HOLY ACTION

1. Stop circular thinking. A labyrinth leads to God. Worry and anxiety go in circles that lead nowhere. When you next catch yourself in the circle of worry, give your anxious thought this simple command: "*Stop.*" Immediately substitute a positive thought. If the worry returns, say again, "*Stop.*" And think a positive thought. By refusing to let worry stay, your emotions will brighten and you'll have more power to handle your actual situation. This technique works. I've used it! When I stop my worry thoughts, I often substitute this prayer: "*I am at peace. My heavenly Father knows what I need.*"

2. Absolutely, positively take breaks. Refuse the kind of pride that thinks, "No one else can do this." Instead, humbly acknowledge that you cannot be God's servant unless you regularly find a little time for yourself. Adopt the idea of "morning minutes" or look for other ten-

minute opportunities you can scatter throughout your day. Make it a habit to leave the sick room on your break, and whatever you do in those few minutes, let it be something just for you, not merely another chore assigned by someone else. Start your break with a murmured, "Thank you, God" as a reminder that God graces your time out.

3. Accept the unknowable. So often, we simply don't know why someone became ill or what purpose suffering has in our lives. Seeking answers to unanswerable questions only wastes time and energy. Who can explain, for instance, why Dana Reeves, Christopher Reeves's widow and a non-smoker, would die of lung cancer, leaving their only son an orphan? Life is a mystery.

4. Our assistant pastor once took a hike in Colorado. On the trail she saw a rock painted with these words: "The mountain doesn't care." Neither, she said, does life care. Rain falls on the just and the unjust. It's not personal. What we can believe is that God cares. And the merciful God will help us find within ourselves the strength, courage and wisdom to handle any situation. Just don't try to figure it all out.

5. Live your prayer. Maybe you can't change the big picture, but you can minister cheerfully to your loved one in small ways, offering each as a prayer-in-action. When an action is done with "right intent," it becomes a blessing instead of a chore. For example, you can:

- Give a back rub
- Spray lavender or chamomile on a pillow as aroma therapy
- Offer ice chips
- Change a dressing
- Comb hair
- Make a bed more comfortable
- Respond to crankiness with compassion.

6. Practice good communication. This is a book about prayer, which is how we communicate with God. There are also certain skills that can help you communicate better with the patient, the doctors, other family members, friends and neighbors and, in some cases, people in the workplace.

   Many caregiver websites offer resources to help you build skills in specific caregiving communications. Also, the Holy Spirit is wonderfully responsive when we pray for inner guidance before tackling potentially troublesome dialogue.

7. Learn about resources. So often the role of caregiver comes without warning. With no preparation, you stumble along, trying to get it all done, not knowing what community resources could lighten your load.

Think of these resources as the body of Christ: all of us acting in concert to aid one another. When a friends asks to help, you might reply, "Please find out for me what local caregiver services exist and get me phone numbers." Some to think about are:

- Lifeline, an electronic medical alert button your loved one can wear to summon help
- Meals on wheels for proper nutrition
- Volunteers who visit shut-ins
- Door to door van-transportation services
- Voluntary telephone reassurance
- Adult day care services
- Homemaker and chore services
- Volunteers to help you navigate insurance paperwork.

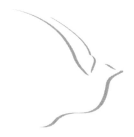

CHAPTER NINE
WHEN ALL IS SAID AND DONE
ONE-MINUTE PRAYERS

You—and every caregiver—truly symbolize the Good Samaritan of the Gospel story (Luke 10:25–37). You did not pass by, but *stopped and took pity*.

And Jesus asked, "Which was the true neighbor?"

"The one who showed mercy," was the reply.

And Jesus said, "Go thou and do likewise."

You are doing just that.

The Compassionate Creator of us all observes when the

gentle touch of your hand brings a smile to someone in pain, and listens as your voice calms a loved one's fear. And God sees your exhaustion, anxiety, and grief as you handle difficult day-to-day situations, often in the face of daunting odds. God is aware of all that you go through.

But I have found that God's strengthening love becomes most visible after we surrender our belief that we are in control of the situation. The greatest challenge and the greatest gift we experience as caregivers is learning to let go, learning to trust in the ultimate good of whatever will be.

Helen was a caregiver to her mother and, several years later, to her husband.

In caring for her mother she became "obsessed," as she put it, neglecting the rest of her family, convinced that if she just tried hard enough, she would be able to wrest her mother free of her cancer. It was not to be.

When her husband became wheelchair-bound through diabetes, Helen began reminding herself daily that he was in God's hands. "Once I realized I was powerless and decided to yield control to God, a terrible burden was lifted from my shoulders. I prayed frequently, but I no longer held myself responsible for the life of another person."[7]

In my mother's final days, I, too, came to a place of surrender. My prayer changed from, "Let my mother live," to an accepting faith that God's love for my mother was even greater than mine, and I could trust in the outcome because whatever occurred, my mom was in God's hands.

I could echo Julian of Norwich, the fourteenth-century Benedictine mystic, who cried out joyfully, even in the face of the Black Plague, "All shall be well, and all shall be well, and all manner of things shall be well."

Jesus also taught that the kingdom of heaven is within, which makes every task in our ordinary day potentially holy if we do it with right intent. Here's how this unfolds in our caregiving tasks. I call these our "one-minute prayers."

Oh Lord, as I count out these pills, *cutting some in half to make it easier to swallow, I am reminded that life brings to each of us problems that seem hard to swallow. But your grace works in ways we do not always understand, and what is hard to swallow now may be medicine for the soul if I am open to the lessons available to me in each experience.*

Oh Lord, as I change these sheets, *I am reminded that wrinkled sheets become painful to sensitive skin when a body must lay on them for some time. And seemingly small actions when continued over time can become large, hurtful habits. Guide me in noticing any small words or deeds of mine that can be hurtful. Give me the strength to stop while they are still small.*

Oh Lord, as I bathe my loved one, *I am reminded of the night Jesus bathed the feet of the apostles and said, "I have set you an example: do for others as I have done for you. No servant is greater than his master." May this act of bathing remind me that every time I do for another, I am also doing for God.*

Oh Lord, I am preparing a meal for someone who has no appetite. *As I look for ways to make food more appetizing, I prayerfully remind myself that I cannot force another to eat any more than You can force us to follow what you know is best for us. Help me to do my best in preparation. Then help me to accept another's choices.*

Oh Lord, as I sit in the waiting room with my loved one, *I am feeling impatient and bored. But in describing what love is, Paul's first word in 1 Cor 13 is "patient." So instead of grousing, I thank you for this opportunity to learn more loving patience. And next time, I'll bring something funny to read or look at to give us both a little laugh while we wait.*

Oh God, as I help my loved one into a wheelchair, *I give thanks for the designs and mobility of all the devices available today to help the disabled. May my loved one see this chair not as a prison, but as a way to live in greater freedom.*

Oh Lord, today we are going for a drive. *My loved one is so excited to see the world outside the sickroom. Sometimes I forget to appreciate the beauty of your natural world. Help me feel the same excited wonder as my loved one feels.*

Oh Lord, as I wearily begin another caregiving task, *I recall what your servant Meister Eckert said: "The way to holiness is to do the next thing you have to do with all your heart* *and soul and with delight." Oh God of light and love, help me to find the delight in this task. If I lighten my attitude, I will feel less weary.*

Oh Lord, the stack of hospital bills and insurance forms is so intimidating. *How will I ever make it through the fine print? I rely on Scripture, which says, "for God all things are possible" (Mark 10:27). All I have to do is breathe, focus, and take it slowly—if not one step, then one word at a time. Thank you, Lord, for helping me in the process.*

Oh Lord, as my loved one convalesces, *guide my imagination in creative ways to make my visits more enjoyable: by reading aloud a well-plotted story, bringing in a pet, sharing photos from family albums, checking out cartoon books from the library, planting seeds in a flower pot, listening to show tunes. . . . Open my mind to possibilities, remembering what Proverbs 17:22 says: "A cheerful heart is a good medicine."*

And finally, oh Lord, thank you for helping me see my caregiving tasks as prayer opportunities, *so that each one becomes a kind of holy experience. With your grace to strengthen and encourage me, I will find the faith to say, as I care for my loved one, "All shall be well, and all shall be well, and all manner of things shall be well."*

Resources

Here are a few of the resources available to caregivers, primarily online.

Cancer Information Service
Toll Free: 1-800-422-6237

CareGivers.com
17 Applegate Ct
Madison, WI 53713
Phone: 608-256-0488
E-mail: support@betteraging.com
Internet: www.caregivers.com
888-405-4242 for an elder care specialist
www.DisabilityInfo.gov

A comprehensive online resource for people with disabilities managed by the U.S. Department of Labor's Office of Disability Employment Policy (ODEP), in partnership with twenty-one other federal agencies.

Eldercare Locator
Administered through the US Administration on Aging.
Toll Free: 1-800-677-1116

Family Caregiver Alliance
Internet: www.caregiver.org
First non-profit community organization to address needs of families providing long term care at home. Established the National Center on Caregiving to advance high quality, cost-effective programs and policies. Offers a state-by-state resource map online.

Hospice Foundation of America
1621 Connecticut Ave., NW, Suite 300
Washington, DC 20009
Toll Free: 1-800-854-3402
Fax: 202-638-5312
E-mail: hfaoffice@hospicefoundation.org

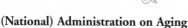

(National) Administration on Aging
Washington, DC 20201
Phone: 202-619-0724
E-mail: Aoainfo@aoa.gov
Internet: www.aoa.gov.

National Family Caregivers Association
Educates, supports, empowers and speaks up for those who
care for loved ones with a chronic illness or disability or the
frailties of old age.
10400 Connecticut Avenue, Suite 500
Kensington, MD 20895-3944
Toll Free: 1-800-896-3650
Phone: 301-942-6430
E-mail: info@thefamilycaregiver.org
Internet: www.nfcacares.org

Today's Caregiver Magazine
3005 Greene St
Hollywood, FL 33020
Toll Free: 1-800-829-2734
E-mail: info@caregiver.com
Your Area Agency on Aging
This resource will be listed in your city or government
sections of the phone book under Aging or Social Services.

Well Spouse Association
63 West Main Street, Suite H, Freehold, NJ 07728
Toll Free: 800-838-0879
Phone: 732-577-8899
E-mail: info@wellspouse.org
Internet: www.wellspouse.org
A national, not-for-profit membership organization which
gives support to wives, husbands, and partners of the
chronically ill and/or disabled. Support groups meet monthly.
Well Spouse publishes a quarterly newsletter, "Mainstay."

NOTES

1. Emily Dickinson, poem number 254, *The Complete Poems of Emily Dickinson*, edited by Thomas H. Johnson (New York: Little, Brown and Co., 1960).
2. This poem by an unknown author is from Henri Nouwen, *With Open Hands* (Notre Dame, Ind.: Ave Maria Press, 1972), 85.
3. Thomas à Kempis, *The Imitation of Christ*, (trans. Richard Witford; New York: Doubleday/Image, 1955), 134.
4. Henri Nouwen, *The Open Hands* (Notre Dame, Ind.: Ave Maria Press, 1979), 82.
5. Rabindranath Tagore, *Show Yourself to My Soul*, trans. James Talgrovic (Notre Dame, IN: Sorin Books, 2002).
6. Teresa of Avila, in John J. Delaney, *Saints for All Seasons* (New York: Galilee Trade, 1979), 128.
7. Adapted from *Vibrant Life*, p. 27, May-June, 1993.